THE
SPIRIT
of PRESENCE

*A Reminder & Guide for Massage Therapists &
Bodyworkers From Beginner to Experienced*

JÉNAL N. MENOLA

BALBOA.
PRESS
A DIVISION OF HAY HOUSE

Balboa Press books may be ordered through booksellers or by contacting:

Balboa Press
A Division of Hay House
1663 Liberty Drive
Bloomington, IN 47403
www.balboapress.com
1 (877) 407-4847

Because of the dynamic nature of the Internet, any web addresses or links contained in this book may have changed since publication and may no longer be valid. The views expressed in this work are solely those of the author and do not necessarily reflect the views of the publisher, and the publisher hereby disclaims any responsibility for them.

The author of this book does not dispense medical advice or prescribe the use of any technique as a form of treatment for physical, emotional, or medical problems without the advice of a physician, either directly or indirectly. The intent of the author is only to offer information of a general nature to help you in your quest for emotional and spiritual well-being. In the event you use any of the information in this book for yourself, which is your constitutional right, the author and the publisher assume no responsibility for your actions.

Any people depicted in stock imagery provided by Thinkstock are models, and such images are being used for illustrative purposes only. Certain stock imagery © Thinkstock.

Print information available on the last page.

ISBN: 978-1-5043-7615-0 (sc)
ISBN: 978-1-5043-7616-7 (e)

Library of Congress Control Number: 2017903242

Balboa Press rev. date: 03/01/2017

To all of the wonderful, magical, and ever-so talented massage therapists and bodyworkers that have crossed my path.

CONTENTS

PREFACE

What a gift it is to be a part of someone's healing journey. As a massage therapist or bodyworker, we are instruments, utilizing our knowledge, our strength, and our compassion for others. I have always been fascinated and thrilled to be a part of this industry. All of us are at different levels of expertise in our practice. Yet we all have a common interest: the desire to help others. Our desire to help others can come from a deep-rooted understanding that we are all connected in this universe. By helping one another, we are actually helping ourselves. The wish to treat others in the way we would like to be treated perpetuates the cycle of "one good deed deserves another." We are all connected as humanity and by the intention of caring for each other and this Earth. By sharing love and compassion, we can create a beautiful environment. And by sharing that love, we can help make this world a better place.

We all share the inner knowing that we have something to offer humanity. We may not be able to place words upon this feeling but we just know deep down inside that we can help. And some of you have chosen to be massage therapists and bodyworkers in order to do your part and offer your care and compassion to the world.

Each one of us has our own story, a story that has led us on a journey to help ourselves, others or both. The reason we have been called to this profession is because massage therapy and bodywork have done something wonderful for us personally. They have touched our lives in some way. Something made us feel so good, so excited, so inspired, that it fueled us with a desire to share it. Or to say "that was so amazing, I want to know how to do this for another, I know I can help." That impact was so strong that we feel compelled to give that to another. To be a part of this wonderful world of massage therapy and bodywork is an honor. What makes this profession so amazing is that the joy it brings you continues to grow. You are always learning and growing in the field and, therefore, in your personal life as well. You will take these experiences as more knowledge to fine tune your intuition for future use. The more you give, the more you will get. With every experience, you will only grow.

At an early age I had decided that I wanted to be an artist. I loved drawing, painting, sketching, crafting, and sculpting. I wasn't great at it, but I was good, and I enjoyed doing it. So naturally, I went into the direction of the arts when it came time to attend college. I started off majoring in graphic design. I didn't think I would find a career in just painting and sketching, so I took an avenue that was a more lucrative option for the long run. I started out taking all of my fine art courses prior to starting the computer art and graphics portion. Once I began my graphics classes, I struggled. I couldn't comprehend the creative thoughts in my mind and convert them onto a computer screen. How could this be? I was an artist. "I can figure this out," I told myself. After continuous effort, I decided it wasn't for me. I chose to drop out of college.

That same week I came across a posting for an introduction to massage therapy class. I was already down on myself for dropping out of school, and this idea had really grabbed my attention. I thought, "What do I have to lose?" So I gave it a try. And this is where I fell in love. This subject just intrigued me, I was excited to show up and learn. My new passion was waiting for me. And it all made sense now. I needed a hands-on approach to my work. I couldn't express my art on a computer screen because I needed to use my hands. I was so thrilled and so in love with my new profession. My life had changed and my journey had only just begun. Little did I know that massage therapy would shift my life and take me around the world. Massage therapy has changed my life forever in the most amazing ways possible, and I continuously give thanks by sharing it with the world.

Words cannot express my passion for massage therapy and bodywork. When you are meant to do something, you can truly feel it in your entire being. The absolute joy that I feel when assisting others on their healing journey cannot be hidden. I know with all my heart I was meant to do this work. When I am present with a client and the session begins, the strong resonance I feel with the work I do cannot be denied. I am meant to do this work.

The Spirit of Presence was written for all my fellow massage therapy and bodyworkers out there, in hopes that we can all continue to grow in this profession together and to expand our love across this universe.

ACKNOWLEDGMENTS

I have had the pleasure and privilege of travelling across the globe doing what I love. I have met and worked with some of the most talented massage therapists and bodyworkers in the world. I am so blessed to have been in their presence. Thank you for the gift of your touch and kindness. You have taught me, challenged me, and shown me much of what I know to this day.

A very special thanks to every client that has been placed before me: thank you for being teachers. And much love and gratitude to my dearest and sweetest Pumpkin, who teaches me patience, compassion, and unconditional love every day.

INTRODUCTION

There must have been some significant experience to lead
you on this path as a massage therapist and/or bodyworker.
Something influenced you to choose a path of helping loved
ones, communities, and humanity, with this specialized gift
and skill. I am here to explain some of the unspoken parts
of being a massage therapist and bodyworker—some things
we all do, yet do not speak about or never think to discuss.
I am offering another perspective here to help explain or to
help you better understand your calling.

There's a lot that cannot be taught in massage school
or in textbooks because it has to come with experience.
Sometimes not even words can describe what we encounter
in this field. Nor can we predict what could happen or
present itself at any moment. You have to get out there and
literally touch someone to experience this.

As therapists, we are educated and specialized with
skills of compassion, strength, and knowledge. But that
wouldn't be anything without the client. Clients give us the
opportunity to exercise our patience and our eager will to
help others. Each client ignites our true calling and passion

by allowing us to offer what we do best. As specialized caretakers, we are skilled to be ready and available for whatever is presented to us. With our clients as our teachers, we have the opportunity to grow with every new client every day. I am grateful for all of the clients that have crossed my path. They have taught me a large portion of what I know. Just by my being present with patience, they have shown me how far compassion and love can go. I have seen how just presence alone can have profound effects on their healing process, and I watch it inspire me in my everyday life.

Every new client we are presented with can open us to a new discovery. A new discovery as in a new illness, a new type of pain, or learning a new treatment or technique along the way. I want to share with you what almost fifteen years of massage therapy and bodywork has taught and shown me. I offer this material as a perspective for others. This is a guidance tool for beginning bodyworkers and maybe resonance for the advanced. What we do as massage therapists and bodyworkers can be very complex but simplified by one word: *presence.* Our presence is key.

In the spirit of presence, we are open. We are neutral, humble, unconditionally loving, and compassionate. We are open to any person in the need of our assistance. *The Spirit of Presence* speaks about what envelops our purpose in the field of massage therapy and bodywork. It expresses the essence of what we do and what we are. We are instruments of guidance for the client's present condition. Each and every one of our sessions is unique and unlike the next, but the consistency in our practice is our presence. In the spirit of presence, we can have many experiences, but our presence is what carries us.

Presence is where the healing process begins. When we offer this space of healing, healing can begin its magic. From there, we apply our skills. Again, people can find comfort in that support and love in your presence. They can find it there to relax, and then your skills can be applied. The comfort of knowing that they are not alone can bring ease to a client. Creating that space of comfort allows the client to unwind. Find peace and trust in your healing practice. Your presence is what you can offer, and this is the basis of our work. If you can offer a loving and trusting comfortable space, your work is all set up for you. This is your stage. Presence sets the stage for your healing practice.

There are some encounters we can have that make us ponder, worry, or cause us to have ill feelings. This book expresses multiple unspoken aspects of this profession. I hope this book can lead you to comfort and relief in knowing you are not alone and that many others in the profession feel and experience similar occurrences. As a collective group of professionals, we can all help each other expand in this field.

Presence is the state of just being: being in the moment, in the love, in the comfort, in the compassion, and in passing no judgment. When holding that space for another's healing, we can learn to hold that presence for ourselves and have compassion with our own process of life. Learning to have patience with ourselves helps to relieve the ego and remind us to just *allow*. Allow life to unfold and find ease with our actions and decisions. We can learn so much from our clients, and as long as we stay present, we can grow. I love being able to grow and expand in my work and life simultaneously. I am so lucky to call massage therapy and bodywork my passion.

Chapter 1

OUR CALLING

We all have callings. We all have our hobbies and personal joys, and some of us are lucky enough to make a living doing something we love. We come from different walks of life, and this career offers so much. There is such a variety of modalities and specialties on which to focus. Some would say that you are born with the skill of a nurturing touch, but I believe that it is the intent behind the touch. If you have the desire to help, it can be felt in your touch. And this is a gift to share. So don't think you have to be born with this healing touch, because it is all about your intention. If you have love in your heart to share, people will feel this through your work.

In this line of work, we set our stage with our presence. Presence is a conscious effort and intent in being available. This is where it all begins. In this crazy world, we can get caught up in life and feel alone and helpless. There truly isn't anything more healing than a reminder that people are there for you, to be that gentle hand that rests on your shoulder to say that it's OK. It's OK to let go. You are safe in this space. We can rush and rush in our busy lives, but when those hands rest upon us, we can finally take a deep breath and remember to let go of all the ridiculousness and allow in what truly matters. We can allow our minds to slow down and our bodies to soften. We can put the brakes on our daily stresses, routines, and on life in general, to just stop for a moment and be present in our body.

The beauty of this profession is that it's open to all: man or woman, creative or intellectual, young or old. You don't have to spend four years in college and create a lifetime of debt to become a massage therapist or a bodyworker. There are so many massage and bodywork schools across the globe. They can offer flexible schedules and affordable tuition. And once you obtain that education, there are so many directions that massage therapy can take you.

It always starts with the basics. You get set up with the proper tools and move on to find your special touch. Then you eventually learn about different modalities. You discover the essence of essential oils or tap into Chinese medicine. Or maybe you choose an avenue of spa treatments to learn and have an interest in the healing properties of other cultures and worldly teachings. It's only a matter of time before you find your niche. Or you can continuously up your game and add more specialties into your toolbox of modalities. That's the thrill of this profession. You can enjoy the ride and just gather skills along the way.

New modalities are always developing in this field. This specialized occupation is constantly progressing and expanding. The sky is not the limit when it comes to specific modalities and skills in bodywork or your opportunities. The more you integrate and add to your menu of skills, the more people you can help and build onto your business. It is such a blessing that continuing education is required for all of us to keep our certifications and licenses in good standings. How fun is it that we can continue to learn new things and expand our skills as a requirement? Being required to take more classes helps break up our routines and teaches us something new. We are learning and growing together, and there are always new concepts and therapies to add to our toolbox.

You may be one of those people who is a good listener, or are you one of those people whose second nature is to be a nurturer? Are you always looking to help any way you can? Maybe you don't even know how you can help in a particular situation but just feel a deep desire to be of assistance and have a concern for all involved. Massage therapists and bodyworkers are a breed of these little helpers trying to makes this earth an even more harmonious place to live. Some have been called to this profession but are not sure why. But along the road of their journey, they have learned so many lessons, and they cannot deny they were on this path for a reason.

Bodyworkers are a breed of nurturers. We care about others' comfort. We are always doing what we can to help someone feel at ease, even outside of work. We are just those extra hospitable people. If you are or want to be part of this industry, be mindful of others who like to take advantage of people like us. You are a loving and caring being, and sometimes people will leach onto your kindness. Be conscious of this possibility. You can always be loving and kind, but don't go above and beyond your capabilities and hurt yourself. Don't let an employer overwork you. Don't let clients cancel on you consistently without penalty. Be a professional. It's always good practice to set up boundaries. Try your best to surround yourself with people who have good intentions and want to celebrate who you are and who appreciate who you are. Avoid the ones that thrive on your joy and want to absorb your lovable energy. You will know this type by how exhausted you are after spending time with them. Be good to yourself. There is no need to hide your love; just don't let others take your sunshine.

We are all beings of love. Love is our true nature as human beings. It is just our desire and true essence as massage therapists and bodyworkers to offer love and care to others in need of it. You may be on your own journey, but there will always be help along that road. And this is what we provide as massage therapist and bodyworkers. A space of healing, at a sacred and safe time, for another to unwind. Our work is all for them to have their own peace for a moment. What a blessing it is to be there for another at this time.

I always try to put myself in another's situation in order to get a feeling for what they may need. I did this in my life prior to becoming a therapist, and it has helped me connect more with my clients. If I had a friend that was dealing with grief or sadness, I would think to myself, "What would I like someone to do for me?" I think this idea of thinking about others drew me to this profession. Yes, this is a subjective point of view, but it also allows us to gain more perspective. For instance, if I have pain and tension in my lower back, I will press my fists right into my SI joint, and I will feel relief. I could try this on another person because it has worked for me before. Or it may not work for another, but it's trial and error and how we learn. Think about what you would like and figure out what could bring ease to that body in discomfort.

Have you ever noticed how much a hug made a difference in your day? Or notice how different you felt after that hug? What about a simple phone call, email, or text message from someone saying "hi" and wishing you well? That kind of simple love and attention can feel so good. So can you imagine how much of an impact our nurturing touch and care is felt by a client? We are that presence and attention for that time being. You never know what another person may be going through. They could have stress on their mind or pain in their heart. Either way, they are to be cared for with the equal compassion and care that you give everyone that comes to you for healing.

It is very important for us to give a sacred space and our undivided attention for any client in need. We can care for anyone in need of nurturing by *just* being present. There are some people out there who do not have a shoulder to cry on, a friend to vent to, or a body to hug when life is rough. We can be there for them as that presence. Sometimes all they need is a space to be themselves and to release emotion.

For example, some women need a little extra love during pregnancy. At some point, some don't feel themselves and may be uncomfortable or emotional. Some pregnant women don't experience any changes like this, and they are the lucky ones! I have given many prenatal massages. Sometimes I felt like the woman seemed uncomfortable and the massage didn't provide any relief. Due to all the pillows and propping and the side lying, I would think they weren't comfortable at all. Well, it took a couple of these sessions to realize that the women were so thrilled with their bodywork, and it had been a while since they have had any relief.

As therapists, we try our best to help our clients feel safe and comfortable. When in doubt. always check in with the client and their comfort levels and pressure. I had one prenatal session with a woman who was eight months pregnant. After the session, I asked her how she felt. She told me that sometimes all she needed was to be able to lie still in a comfortable space, listen to spa music, and have the comfort of a light touch. For her, she found relief in the peace of being able to sit still and have my presence. It is so comforting to know that we can help make someone feel whole again.

No matter what has brought you to this profession, no matter what has happened to you in your past to bring you to this path, what will keep you here is that everlasting loving intent. Truly, we are gifted to be that loving support for another in need, to bring ease to the physical or emotional pain they are experiencing. Carrying compassion, patience, and love for all that come into our paths, we open our doors to all who can find relief in our presence. It is a pleasure to find joy in being there in that space for another person. When you feel this, you know with all your heart that this profession is your calling.

Chapter 2

THE BODY

The body is a sacred vessel. It is the home of our soul. It is something to be honored and respected. Our body is where multiple forces and functions are working together to keep us happy and healthy. The body as a whole, and all the body's parts, are moving forward for the goodness of the individual. Everybody is so specific and unique, so it is to be cared for in its own special way. Our bodies are always functioning with our well-being in mind. But all this depends on how we treat our bodies and if we give it proper nutrients and love in order to function at an optimal level.

We take our bodies everywhere we go. It holds all that we are here and now. Mind, body, and spirit are in the present. Our spirit and mind can transcend, but our body is always here in the physical plane, and it is to be cared for and loved in return for all the good it offers us. To respect the body is to trust it as well and to allow it to guide us to nurture it any way we can.

We must be grateful for those clients who come forth asking for our assistance in the healing of their bodies. The work that we do is so very personal. Each and every one of us is protective of our bodies, and we do our best to make sure we take care of it. It truly is a blessing to be asked to assist in another person's healing process; to be a facilitator of therapy to a body in need is an absolute honor.

Our understanding of body language and assessments sets up our sessions. We can begin this before the client is on the table. By reading the body and making intuitive observations, we can get our first clues as to what may be going on in a client's body. We become in tune with the way it feels and responds. As we grow in our professions, we become very skilled at making body assessments. When you see a person walking, you can observe their gait and make note of where the tension or injury may lie in his or her body. You can get a visual of the symmetry of a client's body as they lie on the massage table. Sometimes, you can find that one hip is higher than the other. When you do your over-the-sheet compressions, you can make note of the density of the body and muscles. How does it spring back to place? Is it resisting? As therapists, we can make a conscious intent to heal a specific area once we find the root of the issue or the target area to relieve once we complete the assessments. The body provides so many wonderful clues on how you can help it. The key is to always listen to the body because it will never lie to you. It only wants you to be well, and it will let you know what it needs for balance and health as long as you are paying attention and listening.

A fascinating subject that we frequently run into in this

field is muscle memory. I am speaking of the emotional and physical trauma that people store in their bodies. Many people do not realize that during traumatic moments in their lives, they actually hold the memory deep inside their bodies. They can hold it in their muscle cells and organ tissues. Now, when I say trauma, it means a moment in life that had a deep impact on us. You cannot measure severity of a life event because it is subjective to the receiver, and it is their experience, their own pain, and it is not to be judged by another.

Let's have a quick biology review to freshen up our knowledge. The entire body is made up of cells right? Billions of cells combined to create individual organs, which then create body systems and tissue, and so forth, to combine and create an entire functioning body system. Each microscopic cell is a body in itself. The cell functions individually like a body; like a whole body system. Each cell has a brain, which is the nucleus. It has multiple organs called organelles. It has mitochondria, which is an organelle that acts as a digestive system for the cell. The cell has many parts that reflect our human body systems and functions but on a microscopic level. It's like a mini body within every cell. When we experience any sort of physical or emotional trauma, our body can store this like a scar, but on a cellular level. And many of you know that if you keep working with a scar by massaging, applying lotions, doing myofascial release, you will begin to see improvement in the visibility of the scar. Not to mention the improvements being made under the surface, which we cannot see yet we can feel. Some trauma we are aware of, and we know where we hold it in our body.

Sometimes that trauma can show up in an unsuspected spot. It depends on where we decide to hold it or carry it. It's like an old memory popping up, but not in the mind: it's recognized in the body first and then sent to the brain. Once it goes to the brain, we start to remember the trauma or experience, and in a way, we relive it. It becomes ignited or active in our present mind. Sometimes we can feel the emotion of that moment or how we felt after that moment. We can feel physical pain or emotional pain at this time when it surfaces. Sometimes, it brings back a certain smell or a particular taste in our mouths. At other times, these could even be the triggers for an emotional release. We can even have laughter and giggles! Regardless how your client releases, just be present and ready to follow the body. Wait for its direction. While having the hands still on an area of the client, we can wait for a release or a direction. Sometimes, a word said, heard, or thought can trigger a release or can stir up the trauma. Bringing the trauma to the surface can be painful, but that is where it shall go in order to be released. In our bodies, we can bury a trauma deep in order to avoid it or to try and completely forget it. If it is a matter that we must face, sooner or later it will show up in our lives whether we recognize it or not. To some it may hurt so badly that they would rather bury it rather than deal with it or even talk about it. We can forget about it for years, and even decades can pass without us even being aware of it or remembering that it has bonded to us all this time. To each his or her own trauma. There is no measure for trauma. Everyone has their own pain. You can never compare one's pain to another, because it's all about the person involved and how the circumstance affected them personally. Pain is pain, and it is not to be measured.

You will get clients with this on occasion. Again, our presence is what can help them. Remember this: the pain is theirs, and their own body and mind will let them know how to deal and to release when they are ready. You, as the bodyworker, are to just be present and provide that safe comfortable space for them. Keep comfortable contact unless they ask you to stop. Honor their space and wishes; it can be a very difficult time for them. Maintain a connection and stay in one place until their body tells you to move on or readjust the hold. Always listen to your client and honor their needs in that space. Sometimes we are rooting for our clients and want their progress more than maybe they even want it. Be conscious of this because this trauma is not ours, and we must honor when they are ready to let go. All we can do is be there for them as that care and support.

There are a few ways that muscle memory can be triggered. Sometimes during very deep tissue work, a deep-rooted trauma can surface. Or it can surface by spending a lot of time in one area and really working at a specific spot. Activating it can bring up some old memories. Increasing the circulation and also elevating the vibration of the energy in that location can all stir this trauma up to the surface if it coincides with a thought the client has or with a memory flash. There are different catalysts for different people for their trauma to surface. It's always specific to the individual and should be handled with extra special care.

To care for another's body is an honor. I like my work to be thorough and customized at most times. It's our intention for the client to receive the most benefit with the time given. At times, you may take the client over the designated time because some bodies take a while to warm up and find comfort. After some time, the client will unwind and loosen. Sometimes, holding a part of the body an extra-long time and giving it your full attention can go a long way. We can take that extra time to massage specific areas that may not get much attention and care, and this can feel so good. For example, taking a moment on each finger or each toe can feel so amazing! Instead of skimming over the area quickly, you can take a moment there and work the attachments. Maybe the knees or the elbows need a little extra love. Our joints can get stressed, and that little bit of extra care can go a long way. Increasing the circulation and pushing that stagnant blood or lymph fluid through can help the body on so many levels. We get comfortable with working the larger muscle groups, but our joints and attachments need that special care as well. That attention to detail and that specific intention can be felt strongly for certain clients, and they will appreciate it. A simple movement like this could make a client just melt and experience bliss even for those few moments.

I believe the act of assisted range of motion exercises could have profound effects on a client. And just think, these are the same movements they can do on their own. Yet with your assistance and their trust in you, you give them space of allowing to flow without fear and protecting the body part. There is an active flow that you and the client create filled with trust. Again, the healing is in allowing and presence. When you have the energy of two individuals working together for a common healing purpose, the results are noticeable and the outcome can be intensified. This is one of my favorite techniques because it's where most of my clients get quick, positive results, and it's fun to work as a team for the greater good of their well-being. Working with the body can be fascinating. It will always show you what it needs, and it always enjoys the extra attention.

There's an unspoken language of the body that massage therapists and bodyworkers learn to read over time. The body teaches us patience and teaches us to listen. It speaks to us when we are working with it, and it guides us. It doesn't use words, but it draws our hands to where it needs attention. This is why I always say the body will always show or tell you what it needs, and it will never lie to you. It only wants goodness for you. Your body is always working to benefit you and allow you to perform at an optimal level as long as you put the right stuff in it and treat it with love and respect.

Our bodies are in constant protection mode throughout our busy days and nights. Some don't even relax while they are sleeping at night due to possible high levels of stress or anxiety. I know you have had those clients who do not know how to relax or think they are relaxed but nope! They are stiff as a board! Their arms are held out straight without any bend or softness to them. They are in constant flex mode as you try and massage the tissue, and it feels almost impossible. I always check in with them during this and remind them to take a nice deep breath, try and relax, and become dead weight. Sometimes it works, sometimes it doesn't, and sometimes their relaxation will only last about five seconds. But there is something to the response you get from a body once you place your hands upon it in a massage session. It almost collapses under your palms and fingers. Your touch can be a breath of fresh air to a body in constant tension and defense. You can actually feel that body melt under your touch.

Over time we will build confidence with our touch and our techniques. There is so much out there to learn. That experience alone will only teach us. It's not like reading the information in a book. It's about the hands-on experience. You can't always put words to feelings, and as massage therapists and bodyworkers, we have to put feelings into words to try to make sense of what we work with on the massage table. We are capable of assisting so many others on their journey of wellness. We do something so unique in the wellness field. Sometimes all the client needs is to relax and have the opportunity to release and unwind; an opportunity for their body to speak up without receiving judgments in return. This is a reminder to just be present. And as the therapist, we just have to show up.

Always be open to the body. It is a magnificent work of art. It will always love us, and it will always continue to teach us.

Chapter 3

THE CLIENT-THERAPIST CONNECTION

What we do as massage therapists and bodyworkers is create a space of comfort. Not only do we touch caringly, but we also feel. When we feel, we are listening to the body of the client. We are being present, assessing, and waiting for the body to guide us and to let us know what it needs. We then provide our knowledge and strength once we know what this specific body requires. Sometimes we are not capable of providing what a person needs, but we certainly can gladly give what we have. We can offer that body a space, a space to unwind and allow any release. We can provide comfort of a safe environment to support that body's imbalance and be present for its needs.

In our world today, things have become fast paced and instant. We have conformed to instant results; quick, efficient touchscreens; and not waiting more than a minute for anything. We have easily forgotten how to have patience and how to allow natural processes. This is especially true with our bodies. We've become detached from our own unconditional love for ourselves. Some of us have forgotten to honor the process of healing and change. Our clients are a lovely reminder to us facilitators that we need to have compassion and patience with our bodies as well.

This is why, when I begin a session, I compress the body over the sheet. I know many of you do this as well. It's a wonderful introduction. It's a way of introducing your touch to the clients and letting their body know that it's OK to relax. At the same time, we are making mental assessments while getting their body prepared to release, if it chooses to do so. We are noting the density and tension of the tissues and how loose or stiff the body may be. We are watching how the body responds to our touch. Can you see if this person is maybe nervous and not relaxed yet? At the same time, we are showing this body that it's OK to trust us and to relax; we are here to help. In this moment, allow the body to become comfortable with your touch. From there, we can assess a body and do what we do best with the information we have. Trust in the process. You will be presented with situations that create experiences from which you will benefit.

Have you ever taken a ballroom dance class or any type of partner dance? In these dances, there is a leader and a follower. The lead, of course, is the person taking the first step and guiding until the end of the song. The follower waits for all direction from the lead. The follower can only go where the lead guides him or her, and he or she waits for every command to move, yet is knowledgeable of the proper steps for the specific dance. I like to refer to this as a very helpful guide for therapists. This is what I use in my massages and bodywork. Many therapists would think that they are the lead, but actually, they are the follower. This is why I begin with the compressions to give an introduction to the space. It is like meeting a person for the first time and shaking his or her hand.

This is familiarizing the client with your touch and presence, which helps him or her to become comfortable and trusting of you. Then there is the application of oil or cream. I consider this the warm-up, and it sets up the space for a comfortable session. As a therapist, you are feeling the textures and tensions and making assessments. You feel the body's temperature, the body's reaction to your touch, and you're making observations of the client's current condition. You are taking the discomforts they have told you about and comparing them to what you are actually feeling. You are also checking the fascia and how the body easily moves or doesn't move, and then you pause and allow the lead, which is the body, to begin.

If nothing is happening, I usually take a moment to ask the client to take a deep breath. This signifies that *we are beginning and I am ready to support you during this release.* The breath work reminds them they are in a safe place to relax and brings them into the present moment.

Have you ever found yourself in the middle of a massage session where you get stuck in one spot, and you stay in this spot and just hold there? When I say hold, I refer to a time when your hands lightly cover a specific area of the client's body, like when we apply a cranial hold and cradle the head in our hands. We use a few grams of pressure and just support and hold the body in this place.

This can actually be done in other areas of the body. You stay there because the body is guiding you to be there. It is the body telling you to be there and stay there until it is ready to release. It's important to stay connected at this time and wait for the lead to continue the dance. It's an intuitive calling made by the body. It's saying, "Please stay with me at this time. I need help getting through this release." And this is what we as therapists are reading through the body. You may not know why you're holding that particular area or what has stopped you, but something brought you to that spot. As therapists, we must learn to trust the body intuition and body talk that happens between client and therapist and to know the difference between listening to a body and listening to our own ego telling us to fix and approach the body differently. Always have the client's best interest in mind. It's key to learn how to differentiate between what the body needs and our own overpowering will to help fix.

At this point in my career, I have approximately worked on over 15,000 different people. That is a lot of bodies and a lot of diversity. Over time, I started to see patterns and recurring conditions. Just like in life, every moment is an opportunity and an experience. Every client that comes to you is a new opportunity. This is an opportunity of knowledge and growth. Every single client that lies on your table is going to teach you something. You will always gain something from an experience with a client, whether it be knowledge, intuition, or strength.. They can teach us to be better listeners and how to be present more authentically.

Always see the good in all that comes to you. Trust in the process that you will be presented with situations and experiences that will only benefit you. You can grow and there is only goodness in growth. At times, there may be negative situations that occur or circumstances where you must decide whether you should make better ethical decisions as a professional, all which will benefit you in the long run. How can we ever learn if we are not faced with these issues and able to learn from our mistakes or experiences? Learning to embrace even the most negative of circumstances is a challenge. But when you realize that it was only put into place to help you, you can then appreciate it.

There is nothing more rewarding than seeing our hard work pay off. Seldom do people get to see their work make a difference in this world, but in our industry, we get to observe this many times. The impact we have on others generates through them and is carried into the world.

Whatever you are presented with—be it clients, illnesses, medical conditions, or ethical decisions, all will only make you experienced and wiser in your profession

Isn't it funny how you can be approached with a certain illness or condition through a client or maybe even in your own personal life, and then all of a sudden it seems like everyone that comes to you has this issue? Coincidence? Or are you being called to better understand this issue for self-healing and helping others? Well, that's what I like to believe. I feel that the better we understand how to care for ourselves, the more we are able to be of more assistance to others in need. This is how we grow into extraordinary bodyworkers.

Being more informed and experienced in understanding body conditions makes us into more successful therapists.

The client-therapist connection is key. As two individuals work together for the greater good of the body's well-being, clearly in this moment only wonderful things can happen. This is where the magic happens. As we further our careers and learn how to read bodies and to connect with the body, we will truly grasp what is best for the individual client. We will also learn how to better assess and to create that space of healing catering to that specific individual. Always keep that connection and listen to their body. This will be your greatest strength as a massage therapist and bodyworker.

Chapter 4

BE THE LOVE, NOT THE EGO

We are not magicians. We are not all-knowing healers. We are facilitators of energy, strength, and care. We are all on that path of learning how to do it better the next time. There are a good number of us that are quite intuitive. Actually, we are all intuitive beings. We just have to practice and fine tune our perceptions to express this gift. We know how to utilize our special skills, which are designed to be beneficial for the human body, and yes, I absolutely agree that there are some people out there who make you feel like you have been dramatically transformed in the most amazing way! Again, it's in the want and desire we have to help others. We are so blessed to be that facilitator of such love. We have our favorites out there; our favorite therapists with "magic hands." Sometimes we can find a therapist that energetically matches our needs and can read our bodies better than we can. Again, the more experience you have, the keener your observations become, and your body intuition will grow. You will be so familiar with body energy that you can possibly find ease in reading your client's body.

At this time, I ask that you put your ego away. Understand that we do not fix people. We assist people in their healing process. We provide a comfortable atmosphere for those in need of relief. We have gained the knowledge and intuition of the healing arts in order to facilitate these services to assist others in need. Everyone is capable of this, but some people are closed off from this and haven't remembered how to express this gift.

As therapists, we learn to tap into something deeper than the surface. We can see beyond what the eyes can see or what they have been trained to see. This isn't magic but a sense or gift that all of humankind holds. We are blessed with opportunities to do this daily in our work. How lucky is it that we massage therapists and bodyworkers can utilize this talent and therefore can use it in our own personal lives? We know how to use our hands to help people find relief. We use our hearts to offer a loving and caring environment. Anyone can do this as long as you want to help others in a positive way and do not have a fear of touch.

But sometimes our egos get in the way. We can feel so strongly that we know what another person needs. Hey, we may know sometimes, but we don't always know for certain. As therapists, we are not certified to give or read MRI or CT Scans. We do not have X-ray vision to explain someone's pain or discomfort.

Learn to differentiate between your ego and intuition. Remember, it's not a quiz, nor is it about getting it right or wrong. It's not about figuring things out for the client and "fixing them." It's not about us trying to prove that we know what's best, because we don't always know. The body knows. We cannot fix anyone. Clients can only fix themselves. We are there to help facilitate this healing process for them. We are with the client on *their* journey.

It's an honor to be asked to facilitate this kind of healing and to join them on this journey by helping guide them into wellness. We can offer what we can. Again, it is our presence that helps pave the way for them to healing. Our presence creates a space for changes to happen with ease and comfort. We are so lucky to be able to do this as our career and profession. What an exciting place and time in humanity to be in!

And we can make mistakes. It's OK. Don't let your ego tell you any differently. Have you ever lost focus during a session and couldn't recall if you massaged a certain area? I know I have done this too! All of a sudden, you are stopped and have a mild panic attack. At this point, I hope the client is asleep and hasn't notice this pause of panic. But I will usually go back and check the body part that is questionable to see if oil or cream was applied. I will add extra compressions to try and make it flow and feel like this was all part of the massage routine. It happens, but what can you do? You make it work and keep the client comfortable. Again, this is a lovely reminder to stay present and focused.

Be humble. We can learn so much from others and our environment. Look at every experience as an opportunity to grow. You do not know all there is to know about massage and bodywork. The field is always expanding and growing. Also it's to be acknowledged that every human being is unique in their chemical, physical and emotional makeup. There is such diversity and complexity out there. Nobody knows everything out there, but with every day and every experience we have, we gain a little more insight and a better idea or understanding of the world around us. The more we open the door to acceptance and embrace life and all of its uncertainties, the easier it will be to drop our egos.

You are not above any other. You have skills just like the next person. Maybe not be the same skills, but they are your skills and talents. Always be in that loving and compassionate space for a client. We don't need to control their situation, because it is not even our situation to control. Some massage therapists and bodyworkers can get frustrated with clients for not taking their advice on a recommended method of wellness. Or they may be frustrated by a lack of commitment to the method of wellness. But you have to understand that it's their body. We can recommend and suggest, but they're the ones with a choice because it is their body, their vessel of life, their choice. And it's our job to be compassionate and honor their decisions.

Have you ever had a client come to you with a condition or pain and you said, "Oh, yes, I know exactly what you need." And once you had them on your table, you realized it wasn't what you thought and what you thought you knew wasn't working. The ego does not like that!

My point here is that you just need to be open and accepting, and truly, we don't know all there is to know about the body or each specific person. If you welcome every person as a clean slate, I guarantee you success. Open mind, open heart, clean slate, without judgment. And allow them to guide you. They know their bodies far better than you do. Whether it's conscious or not, they are far more connected to their bodies than you are to them. Listen to them. Their bodies will inform them first of what feels right.

Again, be humble. Know the difference between what's best for another and what our ego is trying to prove. The ego can convince you that we know what's best for another person, but this is not always the case. We can gladly make suggestions or offer ideas for one another. Anything that the client can do to try to bring themselves comfort will only help later, but they must be willing and open. Never force anything onto them. When things are forced, people can feel intimidated. Sometimes forcing something can extract all the compassion and care from the circumstance. When this happens, it no longer comes from a neutral, peaceful place. It's coming from an ego or a place of control.

And sometimes it works in a reverse manner. At times, you will get a client that comes to you and asks you to "fix me." Truthfully, I cannot fix anyone but myself, but I am happy to offer them my presence. Please ignore the guilt of obligation you may feel when someone asks you to "fix them." Don't feel pressured or obligated. Remember, we are not magicians.

We can provide them with a space of healing. And you don't even have to say anything to them. Just be there. Humor them when they say, "Fix me." I always say, "Let's find you some relief." When I speak to a client about their body, I speak for us both. I will use words like, *let's*, *we*, or *together*. Because combined, client and therapist, we are working toward the client's optimal well-being. It's a team effort.

As much as they may believe they are doing nothing, they are actually allowing the whole process to be. By relaxing and allowing a healing process to take place, the client is what makes the session even possible. By placing their intention on healing, they will influence their own wellness. So just continue to do what you do best and create a special healing space for your clients.

I know many therapists who feel so guilty after a session because they say they wished they could have done a better job or done more to help the client. As long as you were doing your best, there isn't more that you can do. Sometimes their bodies can't handle more. Just honor the process of their body and where the session naturally takes you. It's a beautiful thing that we care so much that we wished their discomfort to disappear. Again, we must remember that the client's pain and discomfort is their own, and it is up to the client how they recover.

Taking on a client's pain as our personal problems can cause issues and conflicts in our own lives. Their pain is not ours. It is not ours to make better or make worse. It's not our call. Their pain is a life lesson for them. Their pain is an experience from which we as therapists grow. It's an experience for us to gain knowledge, but it is never for us to take on as our responsibility.

You never know ever what's in a person's mind or heart. Clients are always welcomed to share, but that doesn't mean they will or want to. So have compassion because you may not know the hardships they are going through. You don't know what they are feeling or experiencing. And this holds true for any encounter in life with another person. Be that presence and loving space for all that come to you.

Remember, if you're doing your best, that's all you can do. No more. Do not put your mind and body in jeopardy. Sometimes there's more going on in a client's life than we can pick up on. Honor that. If we are meant to address what they have going on, then it will present itself. It's not for us to force out of them. Again, our work is in our presence. As long as you are present for them, you are doing exactly what you're called to do. Don't beat yourself up or allow your ego to tell you that you can fix someone. Honor the client, and honor yourself. Be present. Their process and their journey is solely theirs. Just be there in that space and offer them comfort.

Chapter 5

BEING YOUR BEST SELF

Always do no less than your best. Some would think that giving your best means going above and beyond our limits, but that is not true. Giving your best doesn't mean killing yourself physically and psychologically. It means giving the client your undivided attention with the client's best interest in mind, while simultaneously upholding your integrity and well-being. There is no such thing as doing more than your best. Beyond your best becomes overkill, and it's no longer your best, because you are stretching yourself beyond your capacity, which in turn will drain you. You cannot have any feelings of guilt or regret that you could have done more for that person when you've already given your best. End of story. If a client isn't satisfied, just know that you did all that you could, and it is not your fault. Hopefully they will find a therapist out there who can help them, or you can discuss with them their area of disappointment and get a better idea of what you could do the next time. Getting their feedback will help you to find where you can grow. Don't beat yourself up over a dissatisfied customer unless you do know you could have done something more.

If you were aware that you were not your best, then you will understand their unhappiness. Maybe you weren't feeling well, or maybe you had a personal issue on your mind and you were not focused on the client. Don't beat yourself up over it—learn from the experience. Reflect on that session. You may have questioned yourself on whether to do something or not. Reflect and see what your instinct told you to do in the session compared to what you actually did do and what the outcome was with the client.

Sometimes you can get a dissatisfied customer, yet it actually had nothing to do with you. A client could have a personal issue and, unfortunately, you were in the wrong place and become the target of their frustration. Learn not to take these circumstances personally. Practice listening to your clients and to your instinct. Develop a relationship with your instinct and intuition. Learn to properly read it for the best interest of your clients. If your best isn't appreciated or approved, remember, sometimes it can be the client. I always like to tell clients that I can only offer my best. It may not be the best in the world, it may not be better than the therapist down the street, but my best is all I can offer to them. No more than my best can be offered. At this current point in my career, this is my best; this is what I have to offer.

I had a woman come to me one day with a terrible headache. She told me, "It's so terrible, and I have a party I must go to this evening, and I cannot go with this headache."

I gladly fit her into my schedule at the last minute and began to work on her. She proceeded to tell me that it was her husband's work party and that there were going to be many people there she didn't want to converse with. I listened to her and addressed her headache with pressure points, aromatherapy, scalp massage—the works. I pulled out all my tricks. I worked on her for thirty minutes, but she had no relief. So I continued for another thirty minutes. In the end, her headache would not dissipate. She got off the table and thanked me. She had no issue with the massage and wasn't upset that I couldn't bring her relief. I believe she had made her decision in her mind that if she had a headache, she could escape going to this party. She then said, "I guess I cannot go to this party." She left unbothered that my massage had not helped her feel better. Who knows what her reasons were, but my guess was that she needed to go through the motions to justify not going to the party. In my opinion, she did not want to feel better, therefore her headache would not go away. She so badly didn't want to attend the party. Again, this behavior is to be honored by the massage therapist or bodyworker. These were her wishes, whether she decided consciously or unconsciously. Her actions spoke clearly that she didn't want to attend this party.

Luckily, she wasn't upset about the massage not bringing her relief, but I knew I had done my best. If she needed more ammunition to fuel her desire not to be at that party, I hope she found peace in whatever the outcome was that night. Of course, the massage wouldn't help if she wanted to have the headache in the first place. I'll say it again: don't beat yourself up when you cannot provide relief for a client. Sometimes they don't want it. I know: weird, right? We all do it.

If you are ill or under the weather, you are not at your best. You know what I am talking about. When you're fighting the sniffles, you have tissues stuffed up your nostrils during a session so that you're not constantly blowing your nose or rubbing your face with oily hands. Would you want a sick therapist working on you? Put yourself in their shoes and reverse the circumstance.

I know sometimes we do what we have to do because of finances or loyalty. But what if you were the client coming in for some bodywork and your therapist wasn't energetically available, sick, or distracted by personal issues? Our clients pay good money for this treatment. If you're unavailable to them, they are not getting what they paid for. It's something to consider in your practice. By not being connected and in tune and holding your best intention, the client could feel this and be turned off. Whether they consciously notice this or just feel a bit off after their session, this can affect your future with them and your reputation. You may not ever see that client again. Maybe nothing happens at all, and they don't notice any difference. It's a good idea for us as bodyworkers to always be conscious of our current conditions and state of mind. This depends on your integrity though. I personally believe in always putting my best foot forward and always being a professional. In this way, my work will always be consistent. Have pride in the quality of your work. If you know that you're a little off at some point, check yourself. Have a little mental chat with yourself about what is going on in your life or how you are feeling.

Make a conscious effort to acknowledge your condition and make an intention that you do not want this to be felt by the client. Some will say a prayer or a blessing. Some will have a personal ritual of some sort to keep their energy to themselves. I will go into more detail later on these personal rituals or habits that we can use to assist ourselves when we are not on our game.

At the beginning of our careers, we are so fresh to the industry and excited to get out there and experience everything. We can be naïve, but it's OK because we are still students. We are always students, actually, always growing and expanding in this industry. At times, we can be driven by money. Depending on our financial situation, sometimes we can be desperate to make more money, or for some, we never knew we could make so much money doing something we love, and we load up our schedules due to the thrill. For us as bodyworkers, making more money usually means taking on more clients, which means more physical labor for us as the therapist. We may put in the extra hours for the cash without thinking of how it will affect us physically or emotionally. Sometimes we don't even notice how we run ourselves down until it's too late.

Think about what you are offering to a client when you are exhausted or in pain. When you start to notice that you don't have energy for anything else in your life besides your job, it's time to maybe take a break. Or reevaluate your balance of work and play. Easier said than done right? I hear ya! But it's something to consider. Conserving your energy is very important. Remember, your job is just your job. It is not your life. Your job and your life are separate.

You can learn things in life and incorporate those lessons in your job. You can also have experiences in your job that can teach you more about your life. But in the big picture, keep these lives separate. Make sure not to take on more clients than you can handle. Be aware of this on a physical and emotional level. Overwhelming yourself can cause a great deal of unwanted stress or potential injury. When the giver isn't at 100 percent, the receiver can suffer on some level. When you're not feeling 100 percent, focus your energy and give a silent wish or blessing in your mind. Set an intention for your session. "Right now, I am not feeling my best, but you have come to me seeking relief. At this moment, I set the intention to give you the best I can offer at this time." This is what I do because I intend on giving the client what they came for. It's like giving yourself a pep talk and hitting a reset button. You have good intentions, and only goodness comes from that.

Sometimes we can overload on work. At times, our finances can encourage us to pick up extra shifts or hours. Whether it's to pay toward bills, a vacation, or an expensive holiday season, we all have our reasons for wanting more money. Have you ever picked up an extensive amount of extra work shifts? And how many of you regretted it before the work load had even been completed? I have been there too, asking myself, "Why did I agree to work all these days?" Or midway through this extra work period, you become ill and must call in sick, leaving your work place short-handed. Think of yourself and think of others when deciding to load up on extra work. Think about what you are doing to your body, and consider the quality of work the client is receiving. Are you putting your best self out there? And lastly, you wouldn't want to leave your work place short-staffed or needing coworkers to cover you because of your own desperation for money. Be mindful and realistic when taking on extra shifts. Our work is very hard, and we need those periods of rest to refresh the body.

Always honor the body. The body will be good to you as long as you're good to it. Because when we take care of ourselves, it's easier for us to be present in helping others. When we're in balance, it's easy to accept anything that comes our way. Now I want you to know I am not sitting here speaking from some sort of pedestal. I am not perfect, but I am speaking about all of these subjects because I have been there and done it! And many times I have said, "Oh, man, if I knew then what I know now!" I have burned myself out and I have overdone it to make more money. I have also made poor ethical decisions. But all of this has made me more aware, knowledgeable, and successful at this point in my career. It has made me who I am today without any regrets. Because I learned from all those mistakes and came out a stronger and more professional massage therapist and bodyworker.

When you know how to love and respect yourself, you know better how to love and respect others. So take care of yourself and this career will take care of you.

Get bodywork! This is what you do for a living! It is what you preach to your clients! Don't be a hypocrite. Make sure you are taking care of yourself and getting regular massage and bodywork. Receiving is always key to our learning and growing as well. I know that every time I receive bodywork,

I walk away having learned something new—whether it's a new technique or about something to avoid. If something felt uncomfortable to me during the session, I will make a mental note and know not to do that to a client or that some clients may enjoy it, even if I didn't particularly find it enjoyable myself.

Our work environments can be so diverse. Sometimes we work in an environment that is solely run by ourselves, and our only interactions are with our clients. Other times, we can be a part of a large team of therapists and bodyworkers working together. Every situation is different, but having a strong work ethic is a great quality to have and to share.

Good boundaries will take you far too. And setting these boundaries early in your career will help keep you successful. If you create these personal laws and rules early, you will create a very ethical routine and practice. When you install these tools from the beginning. they will eventually become second nature to you, and conflicts can be seldom.

I think we are all familiar with the therapist-client relationship no-no, right? Having any sort of outside relationship with a client, whether it's platonic or romantic, is never a good idea. Have you ever had a quarrel about money with a friend? That's not fun at all, and it can end that friendship quickly. Imagine that with a client! It could get ugly and affect the future of your career or business. Always be professional. You do not need to make friendships or relationships with or through clients. That is what your life outside of work is for. In the rare chance that you feel you must be involved with this client, whether as a friend or in a romantic way, you must simply end the professional relationship. And if the parties involved care that much about the relationship, it will not be an issue to discontinue seeing them as a paying client. I'm not suggesting that you not develop any type of rapport or connection with your clients, because you do need to connect with them and to understand them. But they don't need to know about your personal life. They don't need to know what kind of day or week you're having. Usually, they are polite and inquiring, and I know they care about you, which is why they show concern. But you always want to make their experience about them. Redirect that conversation right back at them. You're the therapist and bodyworker for *them*. If you're having a rough week, it's not for them to know because then they are put in a position and on the spot to have compassion and sympathy for *you*. Any good-natured person would do that of course, but remember, they are coming to us for healing. We have our own friends and family that we can vent to about our situations and our own feelings. Clients do not need to be involved in our lives. They need to be reassured that we are devoted to them, which is why they come to us in the first place.

Always use discretion. Discretion can take you so far in this industry. You have no idea of the possibilities this industry holds for you. When you have strong ethics and are a professional, there will be a demand for a person like yourself. When you have skills and integrity, you are an in-demand therapist. Trust me, people talk, and you only want it to reflect your true positive nature. Always represent your best self. Don't be gossipy with your clients. That session is only for the client, and they can speak about whatever they want. They can gossip, but you are there to listen, be present, and not to chime in. This is their release and how they are choosing to spend the time. Respect that. And whatever may be spoken of during that time, that never leaves that room, unless of course the conversations speaks of illegal acts or is about a person is in danger. Again, in this rare circumstance, use your best judgment. And you're not being rude by not getting involved. You are being respectful whether they realize it at the time or not.

Some of you may find yourselves working on high-profile people and celebrities. They are not to be gossiped about and should be treated no differently from any other client you have on the massage table. Remember, they are coming to you for relief and comfort. Be present as you are with all clients. Respect everyone equally, and it will take you far in your career. Remember, the work we do is an honor.

So speaking of gossip! For those who work in an environment with multiple therapists, I have some suggestions for you on keeping your personal life and work separate. We develop close friendships and bonds with our coworkers, and there's nothing more beautiful than the relationships that we can create there.

How many of you work in an environment with a large group of therapists? People like to talk and have opinions. We also all come from different walks of life. There can be quite a contrast of people working together. It is always best to respect each other in this surrounding, but at times, some stronger personalities can pull us into their personal business. People like to stir the pot sometimes; it creates a momentum to feed their feelings about a situation. It may even have nothing to do with work, but they bring their personal life to work. Some will try to drag you into their negative circle of issues they have with work or with another coworker. If it's something that truly bothers you, that is for you to bring up with your supervisor and address from there. Gossiping will not solve anything. It's only a way for you to find others to help justify your feelings. The more people you get involved, the bigger the tornado of emotion becomes. Think to yourself, would you want this aggravation to turn into a monster of a storm? Or are you seeking a solution? Think about how you want to be treated in this circumstance, and it's totally normal to get frustrated with work. We all do at some point, but how you choose to act on it or not to act on it is your choice. You can complain or bicker about whatever is disturbing you, or you can focus your energy on a resolution. Ask yourself if there is another way to handle things.

Then there are those coworkers who complain no matter what. They will complain they are working too much, and then the next day complain there is not enough work! It's crazy, but I think we have all been there. Sometimes these negative circumstances create an uncomfortable environment for others. I like to always remain focused on why I am there in the first place. I am there to be a peaceful presence for those wanting healing. Remember that everybody that has come to you has come to you with reason and purpose. I trust that the universe brings me only experiences that will help me grow as a professional in this field because when I am in that room doing what I do best, nothing else matters.

When you are being affected by the drama in the work place, remember you have a choice either to get involved or center your focus back onto your purpose. It's extra helpful to have a management team that can easily be available to therapists if there is any issue. Having across-the-board fairness and an open-door policy is important in any work environment. Equal treatment makes a pleasant and fair environment to be in. This will bring longevity to the business and the practice of therapists. In a team environment it's hard to keep everyone happy but if you can make the majority happy then it's the best you can do.

Separating life and work is a healthy mentality and a chore. I say chore because it's not easy sometimes. It takes a lot of work to control that boundary. Some days we can find ourselves frustrated or sad and bothered by something in our personal life. And as badly as you want that issue to go away, it won't magically disappear before we walk into work unless you make that conscious decision to let it go for the time being and readdress it in your personal time. Remember, we are creating a space of peace and healing for others. How can we offer peace and healing if we are radiating frustrations or feelings of sadness from our being? That is not practicing at your best. Ideally, it would be best to sort these issues before going to work, but we all know we're not always that capable. Pending the troubling circumstance, it may just be unescapable. In that case, it may be a consideration to call in sick.

Many therapists have different routines or practices in separating the work and personal life to create that peaceful space. Some like to say a mantra on the way into work or prior to entering the place of business. Some create an imaginary storage box right outside work. You can mentally leave the energy from the circumstance in there before entering work. You know that when you leave for the day, you can pick it up on your way out.

I found that if the circumstance is so intense and I cannot get it out of my brain while working, I will adjust my focus. As I am massaging the body, I will speak to myself in my mind about what I am actively doing in the present moment. For example, my mind is racing on a troubling circumstance. In my mind, I will tell myself, "You can put this issue aside. Right now, you are to focus on this body in need." From there. I will focus directly on a body part, and I will have a dialogue in my mind about what I am doing. I will verbalize in my mind how the body part feels. I will name different muscles that I am palpating. I will name the attachment and origin and note how the body part feels when I do a certain technique. I will do all I can in my mind to maintain the focus on that client and not on my own personal issues. Honestly, it's whatever works best for the individual. This technique has always worked best for my sessions when I have been consumed with a troubling thought.

Learning to separate the personal from work can be easy if you always bring yourself back to intention. For me, my personal life disappears the moment I shake the hand of my client. I have gotten myself into a routine of greeting my client in a way to indicate that this is their time and that they have my undivided attention. The trick is to continue to maintain that focus. I know sometimes in that low-lit massage room, our minds can wander off into another place. It's important to refocus on the present and give our undivided attention to the client.

It is also very important to use proper verbiage. We are not doctors, and we can get into trouble if we choose our words poorly. As you know, diagnosing a person is illegal for a massage therapist or bodyworker. And there are numerous times that clients will be probing you to tell them what is wrong with them. When it comes to soft tissue, we are experts, but again we cannot diagnose. Massage school does not certify us as MRI and X-ray technicians, therefore we really cannot diagnose without some sort of radiograph. We can most certainly suggest to our clients the possibilities of what may be occurring with their bodies. We can suggest in a very roundabout way and always encourage them to seek a professional opinion and care if something is very concerning to them. And always be sensitive to their concerns. We do not want to scare them with false ideas of what could be when all could be nothing at all. So choose your words wisely, and speak with an open mind. We can suggest options for therapies and techniques for our clients, but more than anything, you want to just listen to your client. Use caution, even though we may have good intentions and want to help we can put ourselves at risk. Anyone can come back and accuse us of diagnosing them or misinforming them. It's always wise to just be neutral.

We also want to speak clearly about the therapies we are about to perform or when suggesting a therapy that we offer. When we are clear and concise, we don't leave any space for misunderstandings, and always leave time for questions. Always be open to questions and concerns from the client. Even be clear about how you want the client to position themselves on the massage table. I cannot tell you how many times a person has told me that they have had a massage before, and when I walk into the room to begin, they are so confused how to lay on the table. So to save time and embarrassment. I like to always add how I want them positioned prior to the massage, no matter how many times I have seen this client.

Also, it's very professional to be clear and informed with your client. When we can provide the client with an abundance of information and possibilities, we can do this without it being direct and personal.

Be your best, be clear, and always be professional. At all times, be on your game to the best of your ability. What is your personal moral code? Stand by your words and your work. Take pride in what you do, and honor it always. When people are happy, it always reflects in their work and their passions. Show the world your passion!

Chapter 6

SELF-CARE AND LONGEVITY

It is inevitable that one day we will no longer practice our passion. But until then, we can do all we can to better prepare and make better choices to add longevity to our career.

Having integrity and treating others in the way you want to be treated can add longevity to your career. It can mold you into being an honest person and a pleasant person to be around. Making life enjoyable for yourself, your coworkers, and your clients creates an overall pleasant environment. Give the massage you would want to receive, and take pride in your work, and work will always reward you. Whether it's a smile, a gratuity, a referral, or a compliment, it's always a pleasure to know that your hard work is appreciated.

Our work is so gratifying. I mean, how many people out there get the responses and encouragement that we get from clients? When we're finished for the day, our clients compliment us, and they usually leave happier than when they arrived and even more balanced than before. As a massage therapist and bodyworker, it is highly suggested that you get massaged often, learn new techniques, and get off your routine. Self-work is where the true healing happens and knowledge is gained. By getting regular bodywork, you can experience it yourself and better understand how to offer that to another. As mentioned before, that's the beauty of the work we do. We help others so that we can help ourselves. Anytime I get bodywork done, I of course enjoy it and allow my body to restore itself, but I also make note of things that other massage therapists and bodyworkers do that feel good because some of my clients may enjoy that or could benefit from what I have experienced. Try to make mental notes of the things you like and see how your clients respond. Also make note of the things you don't like.

For example, I went for a massage and the therapist had me lie supine, and she undraped my entire left side. No private areas were exposed, but she wanted to use long, full body stokes. This always feels nice. I did enjoy the long, full body strokes, but when she then began to focus on one part of the body, she left the entire side undraped, and I became cold. So here I made a note not to do this to my clients. Or, if I did this method myself, I would re-drape the client after completing the long, full body strokes. The long, fluid stokes feel amazing and creates a nice flow from the feet to the hips and then up to the shoulder to flow down the arm. This was an excellent experience for me to better know how to care for my clients. The key to growth is experience. As much as our hands-on experience is vital to our growth in the industry, our receiving of bodywork is just as important.

When we humble ourselves and become a student again, we remain open-minded.

Take pride in your work. Honor your work, and you will always be rewarded.

Keep up with your education. It's great that it is required that we complete a certain number of continuing education credits for our certificates and licenses. The more we educate ourselves, the more we can expand our business and offer more to clients.

In the long term, we get better and better at what we do. The more modalities you get under your belt, the more you can offer, and this can increase your salary. Every couple of years, you can raise your rates and add different treatments. If you're at a point of not wanting to add more clients but want to make more money, you have options. Again, learn new tricks and get more gratuities. Learn a new modality that is a more expensive therapy per session. So instead of adding time, you're adding more money to your existing work time. Add enhancements to your services. Offer people aromatherapy or personalized blends of oils. Add foot scrubs, anti-cellulite treatments. There are so many ways you can create this longevity and growth in your career. If you are wishing to add more clients, take a few marketing classes. Learn how to boost your career and boost sales. There are so many classes you can take and can even be used as part of your required continuing education courses. Use the system to your advantage. It's all put into place for your benefit. Expose yourself to opportunity and you will only grow and shine.

Also, take care of your body! I saw a therapist who only

lasted two years in the industry because she had to have so many wrist surgeries. Care for all aspects. Each and every one of us has a unique body, and the special care is specific to every one of us. The repetitive motion and physical stress we endure daily will wear us down over time, in some more than others. It's great to be conscious of this from the start of our career before it's too late to repair. Use your whole body. Learn other modalities where you can use your feet instead of your hands. Use proper body mechanics and be conscious of your movements. You have so many options. Do what you can to make this career easier for you to do what you can to continue the work you love.

Hydrotherapy is great to do for bodyworkers. Soaking the wrists and hands in cold water feels so good after a long day of work and takes down some of that inflammation. Rotating the use of ice and heat on our achy bodies can bring us much relief. We preach this all day to our clients, and hopefully we all practice what we preach and take that time for our own self-care. Using herbal pain relief and anti-inflammatory salves or lotions is easy to do before bed or throughout your work shift. Soaking in a bath tub of sea salts and diluted essential oils can be so relaxing and soothing for the entire body. This will help clear us from the work day and cleanse us. This is a great way to disconnect from our work and be focused on ourselves once we complete work for the day.

A salt rinse is a wonderful form of detachment from the unwanted energies we may have accumulated throughout the work day. Clear all those clients out of your energy and focus the time solely on your self-care. Go to a fitness class that makes you feel good. Keep that body in shape to perform bodywork. Sweat out what you do not need. We need to stay strong and flexible to do what we do all day. Keep that blood and oxygen flowing throughout your system. Increase that circulation and keep your system active and functioning at an optimal level. Try yoga, try tai chi, try meditation, or things that just feel good to your specific body and do what helps you feel stronger. Maybe take long walks outside, enjoy the fresh air, and get the blood pumping through the system. Standing outside in a strong fresh breeze is a great way to cleanse the energies. Imagine that breeze grabbing the unwanted energies from your being and taking them all away to leave you fresh and balanced.

Do not forget about what you put inside your body. Some foods will cause more inflammation in the body. Some foods can make us feel heavy and sluggish while others could energize us! Watch your diet habits and take your supplements. Supplements that will keep you energized and will help maintain strong joints can be beneficial for the work we do. Be sure to fuel the body. Give it what it needs. It will only benefit you in the long run. Be certain to always stay well hydrated. Our work is very physical. Do not forget that. Remember, we can do one-to-two hour sessions at a time and that is a nonstop activity, not to mention how many you plan to do each day. Give yourself some credit. Our work is hard, but we can make it easier for ourselves if we take care of our bodies. So speak with your physician about the proper diet and supplements that will suit your specific body and find what feels right so that you can feel more balanced and offer that presence to another in the best of your ability.

Many of us massage therapists and bodyworks have our own "protection rituals." We each have our own way of preparing ourselves to be in close contact of another person's energy, and we safely put a guard up to keep our own personal energies and space undisturbed by what some client may bring to the table. Remember it is theirs, not ours. A client can bring in a load of negative energy or just uneasy energy that is not for us to take on. Create a safe space for them to unload, yet do not take any of that into your space. Everyone has this at some time, and they are not bad people for having this because we all have it. But it is solely for the owner and nobody else. But again, we create a space for them to release this type of energy, and it is wise for us to know what to do with this energy and how to properly dispose of it. We can cause a lot of harm to our bodies and minds by taking on another's negative and unwanted unhealthy energies. We don't do it intentionally. We do it by caring about their well-being, and we want to do what we can to take away their pain. But we must remember that it's not ours to even take away. It's for them to release when they are ready and when released. It is to be disposed of, not recollected.

An example of a practitioner taking on energy would be a scenario where you take your work home with you. Say you go home after a day of work and you're going about your business but you are thinking about a client you saw that day and maybe thinking about their current situation and what you could say to them next time or how you could help them in the next session. This is OK if it's brief, but if it's consuming you and you find yourself speaking to others about it and creating a momentum of thoughts about someone else, then this has gone beyond your ethical practice. And speaking to others about clients is definitely against our ethics, as we like to keep all sessions confidential and discreet. But you can speak of someone and not disclose their identity. In this circumstance, you are consumed with this person's situation. That is their energy not yours. Let it go. You have done all you could in that moment of their session, and if they need more, they can come back to you for a following appointment. It is not for you to worry about or to fix. Of course, we care, but you have yourself and your life. Sessions are for your clients. Life is for you. There's a difference between taking on energy and focusing on the individual client. You can surrender yourself as an instrument, but do not let in any harmful energies. Devote your energies with intention. There are other examples of when you take on people's energy, but this is a wonderful example that we can all relate to in our work. So create an awareness and find your own personal protection ritual or meditation to get you refocused on you and not on anybody's personal junk. If you haven't found your personal protection ritual yet, I am going to name a few. Maybe you can find a practice to help keep your energies and space safe and healthy. Some people hold on to the energies for a deeper purpose unknown to us and possibly unknown to them as well. Respect that, and always honor their process.

We have our own practices of presence. We have our special rituals to set us up and our own energy-clearing cleanses. For example, I imagine myself in a violet-colored bubble that protects me from others energies. I find peace in this color, and it creates a blanket of safety around me. I know that in my mind and in my heart this protects me and keeps me focused on my practice. It keeps me present and confident in knowing I can offer what I know to that client and finish that session feeling myself and feeling safe. Some can imagine a blanket wrapped around their body for protection. I know of therapists that center themselves before the session and say a short blessing or prayer to keep them healthy and safe as they practice their presence.

Thoroughly cleaning all your equipment is a great cleansing method and a sanitary practice. The client's germs and energies can cling not only you but to your tools as well. Be sure to wipe those bottles with hot soapy water or sanitizing solution. Sanitize those sheets, the massage table, and countertops and surfaces. We wash our hands so much in one day, but be sure to scrub all the way up those arms with soap and hot water. Besides picking up energy, you will not want to pick up any sickness or germs.

Presence is a conscious effort and intent in being available.

Along this wonderful journey as massage therapists and bodyworkers, we grow stronger and keep gaining knowledge. We practice our presence and consciously make the commitment to be good to ourselves so that we can be available to one another. We continue to better understand the human body and how we can continue to make this world a better place by assisting in relieving the pain of others. In doing so, we help ourselves on our own paths.

In all, we are doing our part to make this world a more

joyous place to be. We find joy in what we do, and those who come into our paths find that joy as well. We give and we get in this gratifying work we do. Each and every one of us is out there spreading the love and joy of the healing arts. Let your compassion and care be felt with your special touch. Remind others that they are not alone. There will always be helping and healing hands to ease another. We are that presence of ease and comfort. With every single body you encounter, you share a piece of your gift of compassion, and that can flow onto the next person and on to the next person.

I am grateful for all of you massage therapists and bodyworkers out there contributing to this field. Your compassion and care are not only contributing to the growth of the profession but to the growth and expansion of humanity. Your love and care stretch far and beyond. Keep adding to that domino effect of love and gratitude in this universe. You are so loved. You are love. In the spirit of presence, you are a gift to this universe. Thank you for all your hard work and commitment to the love of humanity.